MANUAL FOR ANTENATAL AND POSTNATAL CARE

An Easy-to-Read Guide to Giving Your Baby the Very Best throughout Pregnancy, Birth, and infancy

BY

KIBOKO FRANÇOISE MACHOZI

I0426336

All rights reserved. No part of this book can be reproduced, transmitted by any means or in any form, or stored in a retrieval system without prior written consent of the author.

www.savelife.co.za

Contents

3

Introduction

As a pregnant woman, your life has become even more special as you are not only caring for yourself, but everything you do now affects your growing baby too. The choices you make and the actions you take affect your baby in positive or negative ways. For this reason you must have sufficient knowledge about what is going on inside and outside of your body so that you may take proper care of yourself and preserve the life of your growing baby during pregnancy.

Child care does not start at the time a woman delivers a child; it starts before she ever conceives, and it must continue from infancy to the time when a child becomes an independent adult.

In this book we will focus on care during pregnancy and birth and child care throughout the baby's first year of life.

Part 1: Care Before and During Pregnancy

If you plan to have a child, it is recommended that you first consult a medical practitioner before becoming pregnant.

The purpose of this consultation is to do a general checkup and perform some blood tests to exclude any diseases or abnormalities that may disturb normal conception or growth of an embryo in the womb.

Some vaccines may be given before you conceive, while others may be given during pregnancy.

Also, a woman wanting to conceive is advised to take 400 mcg of folic acid on a daily basis from the day she plans to conceive and during her pregnancy as well. See *The Importance of Taking a Prenatal Supplement* for more information.

In the following sections, we will discuss immunizations needed before and during pregnancy, what to expect during your regular doctor visits throughout your pregnancy, the importance of taking a prenatal supplement, diet and exercise during pregnancy and foods to avoid, drugs and pregnancy, how to deal with miscarriage, common symptoms of pregnancy, complications of pregnancy, and what you'll need to pack in the maternity bag you take to the hospital.

Immunizations Before and During Pregnancy

The immunization calendar is different among different countries, but the common vaccinations that may be given during pregnancy are as follows:

- Flu
- Tetanus
- Hepatitis B

Other vaccines must be given at least two months before a woman conceives as they may lead to life-threatening disease if given during pregnancy.
Some of these vaccines include the following:

- Rubella
- Measles and mumps Varicella[i]

What to Expect during Doctor Visits

During your pregnancy you should meet with your doctor at least once every month until the time that you deliver and then six weeks following your delivery date.

During these visits your doctor will check different parameters to see that the baby inside your tummy is growing and developing properly.

If you ever notice or feel anything abnormal or troublesome with your body during your pregnancy, make sure to mention those concerns to your doctor during your regular visits.

Counseling will be done during your regular doctor visits, and this is the time for you to ask questions about how to deal with any problems encountered during your pregnancy as well as during the breast-feeding period.

Six weeks after you deliver, your body will have, for the most part, regained its status before you became pregnant. At this time you will visit your doctor for a regular checkup just to make sure that everything is well. At this time you and your doctor may discuss your beginning a contraceptive method.

Common Tests during Pregnancy

- Your weight is measured at each doctor's visit to detect obesity and to find out if your monthly weight increase is within the normal range.

  The monthly weight increase of a pregnant woman must not exceed 1 kg.

- Your height is measured to evaluate if you may need a Cesarean section (also known as a C-section) at delivery time. When a woman's height is less than 1.5 m, it may be difficult for her to deliver naturally as the size of her pelvis may also be small. In such cases a doctor may request some other measurements to determine if she will be able to deliver naturally, and if not a C-section will be planned.

- Blood pressure is measured to detect and treat hypertension as it may compromise the life of both the mother and the fetus. Early detection and treatment of high blood pressure is essential to a healthy pregnancy.

- A urine test is done to detect the presence of proteins (that can signal kidney failure) and sugar (that can signal diabetes mellitus) in the urine.

- While you may experience swelling in your legs throughout pregnancy, especially during your third trimester, your doctor will examine any leg swelling and keep it in check as too much swelling may be a signal of edema (a common sign of kidney failure).

- Your hemoglobin level will be checked to make sure that you are producing enough blood as pregnancy requires a sufficient blood supply for you and for baby.

During your first visit, your doctor will draw blood to determine your blood type and Rh (Rhesus) factor.

The Rh factor is a protein found on the surface of most people's red blood cells. If you have the Rh factor (and 85 percent of people do), your status is Rh-positive. If you don't have it (and 15 percent of people do not), you are Rh-negative.

Note: The Rh factor is not a disease, and it is not contagious; having it or not simply depends on the nature of an individual.

If you're Rh-negative and your husband is Rh-positive, your baby may be either Rh-positive or Rh-negative.

If you're Rh-negative, it's likely that your blood is incompatible with your baby's blood, which is most likely Rh-positive. Rh incompatibility isn't likely to harm you or your baby during your first pregnancy since your immune system is not yet alerted. However, the dangers lies in that if your baby's blood leaks into yours, your immune system will start producing antibodies against the Rh-positive blood, and the next time you become pregnant with an Rh-positive baby, then those antibodies can attack that baby's blood.

Therefore, if you're Rh-negative, your doctor will give you an injection of a drug called Rh immune globulin sometime between twenty-eight and thirty weeks of your pregnancy and then again within seventy-two hours after giving birth. (This second injection is done only if your baby is Rh-positive). This will prohibit your immune system from producing antibodies that may affect your second pregnancy.[ii]

In a case of hemorrhage during pregnancy (after twenty weeks), the injection will be repeated every six weeks.

Note: If not treated Rhesus disease may lead to stillbirth, cerebral palsy, blindness, death, and learning difficulties.[iii]

- An indirect Coombs test may be performed on a pregnant woman to detect the presence of antibodies that may cause hemolytic disease in the newborn.

- You will also be screened for Hepatitis B, HIV, syphilis, rubella, sickle-cell anemia, and thalassemia.

An HIV test will be performed during your first visit and again after two months. In some cases the test may be repeated several times. If you test positive for HIV, you will be submitted to antiretroviral therapy (ART), which will protect your baby from the disease.

The syphilis screening (known as RPR) will take place during your first doctor's visit and later.

When testing for sickle-cell anemia and thalassemia, some medications may be given according to your blood result.

The Importance of Taking a Prenatal Supplement

In order to make sure that you and your growing baby are getting the right amount of nutrients during pregnancy, talk with your doctor about taking a prenatal vitamin and mineral supplement that contains folic acid, vitamin B6, and vitamin D as these are always recommended. The other supplements listed here are also recommended but should only be taken if directed by your doctor.

1. **Folic acid**: For the baby, folic acid prevents brain and other spinal cord defects (such as spina bifida).

   For the mother, taking folic acid protects from cancer and stroke.

   You should begin taking folic acid before you begin trying to conceive, and you should continue taking it until the end of breast-feeding. Ideally, you should begin taking folic acid at least six months before trying to conceive.

   The recommended doses for taking folic acid before, during, and after pregnancy are as follows:

   - Before pregnancy until three months of pregnancy: 400 micrograms per day.
   - From four months into pregnancy until the end of pregnancy: 600 micrograms per day.
   - While breast-feeding: 500 micrograms per day.[iv]

2. **Iron**: Iron develops the muscles of both the mother and the baby, and it prevents anemia.

   Usually an obstetrician/gynecologist prescribes 350 mg of $FeSO_4$ to pregnant women as they need more iron to respond to their baby's needs; however, $FeSO_4$ should only be taken as prescribed by a doctor as it may be harmful for the unborn child.

What to keep in mind while taking an iron supplement:

- FeSO4 must not be taken together with coffee, tea, eggs, or milk as its absorption will be decreased.
- FeSO4 absorption increases if it is taken together with food or vitamin C.
- FeSO4 may darken stools, and it may cause constipation or diarrhea for some individuals.[v]

3. **Vitamin B6** is given to treat nausea and to prevent vomiting as a result of morning sickness.

4. **Calcium and Vitamin D**: A supplement of calcium and vitamin D is given to build up the baby's bones; to prevent bone decalcification of bones in the mother; and to maintain the mother's nervous, circulatory, and muscular systems. Calcium may only be given if requested by your doctor as there is generally enough calcium in your normal diet.

Vitamin D regulates the levels of calcium and phosphate in the body. It helps fight infections and reduces the risk of some cancers, diabetes, and *sclerosis.*[vi]

5. **Omega-3** (Docosahexaenoic acid) promotes healthy development of the baby's brain and eyes but should only be taken if requested by your gynecologist.

Diet and Exercise during Pregnancy

While you are pregnant, you should eat regular well-balanced meals in small quantities and exercise regularly. Keep in mind that eating well does not mean increasing the quantity of food you eat but simply increasing the quality.

Fruits and vegetables contain a sufficient amount of vitamins, minerals, and fibers. Eating at least five fruits of different color per day is helpful.[vii]

Eat foods rich in protein to build up the infant's growing body. Take in plenty of carbohydrates to supply yourself with energy; otherwise, your body will obtain energy from fats, which will produce *ketone* and lead to headache, nausea, and bad breath. Foods rich in folic acid, iron, and other minerals should be consumed to prevent anemia. It is important to consume foods rich in calcium, especially around the third trimester of pregnancy, because the baby is busy building up his or her skeleton. Some calcium-rich foods include broccoli, salmon, almonds, and low-fat milk, for example.

Foods rich in vitamins and antioxidants help your body to get rid of all free radicals and to prevent oxidation.

16

Foods rich in fiber help to get rid of toxins within the body and to prevent constipation.

Foods to Avoid during Pregnancy

During pregnancy make sure to avoid the following foods:

- Raw seafood
- Raw meat (risk of *toxoplasmosis*)
- Deli meat (risk of *listeriosis*)
- Unpasteurized milk
- Cheese made from unpasteurized milk
- Fish with mercury, as mercury damages the brain and delays a baby's development
    - Swordfish
    - Shark
    - King mackerel
    - Tilefish
    - Chunk
    - Tuna
    - Smoked seafood
    - Fish exposed to industrial pollution
- Raw eggs
- Refrigerated meat spread
- Caffeine
- Unwashed vegetables[viii]

It is recommended that you exercise three to four times a week for thirty to forty minutes per day. Exercise will build up your muscles and allow for an easier delivery. Regular exercise will also ease backaches and leg pain that occur during pregnancy and will decrease blood pressure and blood sugar. Exercising will give you energy, reduce constipation, relax your mind, and help you release stress.

Keep in mind, however, that only certain exercises are suitable for your condition.

Before joining a gym program, consult with your doctor to find out if the program is safe and what kinds of exercises you can safely do.

Swimming and marching are better exercises for pregnant women.

Avoid exercising when you are hungry as this may compromise your own health and harm your growing baby.

Always make sure to drink plenty of water before, during, and after exercising.

Stop exercising immediately if you notice any of following signs:

- Vaginal bleeding
- Shortness of breath prior to exercise
- Dizziness

- Headache
- Chest pain

Note: Pregnant women suffering from heart diseases, lung diseases, preeclampsia, cervical incompetency, and premature rupture of membranes must not exercise unless recommended by their doctors.[ix]

Drugs and Pregnancy

Pregnant women must avoid auto medication.
If you are taking medication for a chronic condition, you should inform your medical practitioner before trying to conceive or during the first month you miss your period.

Your doctor will determine if there is any danger for you to continue with your medication while pregnant. If there is a danger to continue taking your usual medication while pregnant, your doctor may change the medication or simply stop it and place you under certain disciplines to avoid the worst.

For example, if you are diabetic, your doctor may stop the antidiabetic drugs you are currently taking and replace them with insulin, or your doctor may simply place you on a particular diet.

There are drugs that may safely be taken during pregnancy, but there are others that may not be safe for the developing infant.

Aspirin, for example, must not be taken during pregnancy at any time.

Other drugs may be taken during the first trimester of pregnancy but not during the second or third trimesters. For example, tetracycline may be taken during the first trimester of pregnancy but not at any other time.

On the other hand, some medications may not be taken at the beginning of the pregnancy or at the end but may be taken during the second trimester. For example, thiazide must not be taken during the first or last trimesters of pregnancy.

If you desire to buy any drugs from the pharmacy, you will have to inform the pharmacist that you are pregnant.

Note: Your doctor is the one who will see which medications are good for you and which ones are not. Rely on your doctor's prescription.

Dealing with Miscarriage

Miscarriage, or spontaneous abortion, is the loss of pregnancy in the first twenty weeks.

Fifty percent of women lose their pregnancies before they realize that they are pregnant. They only notice that their menstruation is delayed and is heavy.

There is a high risk of miscarriage between twelve and fourteen weeks of pregnancy. At this stage hormonal problems can occur as the ovaries decrease their production of hormones and the placenta begins producing them instead. The condition of the internal layer of the uterus at the time the baby is implanted may affect the development of the placenta as well as hormonal secretion. Fourteen to 20 percent of pregnant women lose their pregnancies during this period.

The diagnosis of miscarriage is made clinically.

Note: A pregnancy test will still be positive despite miscarriage until ten to twelve days after miscarriage due to the presence of pregnancy hormones that are still in a woman's system.

Causes

The causes of miscarriage are not well known, but it is thought that the following conditions could cause miscarriage in some cases:

- Abnormality of the embryo
- Progesterone deficiency
- Maternal antibodies
- Teratogens
- Infections like syphilis, chlamydia, or other sexually transmitted diseases (STDs).
- Urinary infection
- Womb infection
- Small womb

- Fever
- Alcohol and/or tobacco use
- Recreational drugs

Warning Signs

The following are the most common warning signs of miscarriage. Please do not delay in consulting your doctor if you notice any of these signs:

- Lower abdominal pain
- Lower back pain
- Abnormal vaginal discharge
- Vaginal bleeding

Prevention

Miscarriage may not be able to be prevented, but there are some measures you can take to decrease your risk of miscarriage:

- Keeping a positive attitude and avoiding stress
- Getting plenty of rest and relaxation time
- Maintaining a healthy, well-balanced diet
- Exercising
- Stopping tobacco and alcohol use
- Taking folic acid
- Visiting an antenatal care service at least once a month
- Avoiding auto medication

Consult your medical practitioner at the first sign of even a minor abnormality with your body; do not wait for the situation to become worse.

Common Symptoms of Pregnancy

Morning Sickness

Morning sickness is the nausea and vomiting that pregnant women experience during the first three months of their pregnancies.

Ways to Reduce Morning Sickness

To alleviate morning sickness, try any of the following methods:

- Eat small portions of food little by little in order to avoid being too hungry or too full
- Avoid drinking while eating
- Drink enough fluids but little by little until you reach two liters at the end of the day
- Drink hot soup, tea, lemonade, and juices
- Eat toast or crackers
- Avoid too many oils or fats
- Take a daily dose of vitamin B6
- Use peppermint essential oil
- Drink ginger tea four times a day[x]

Fatigue

Fatigue is common during the first and last trimesters of pregnancy, but in some cases it may be permanent throughout the whole pregnancy.

Causes

The increased volume of blood pumped by your heart raises your heart rate; as a consequence, you will experience tiredness.

Your baby uses your own energy to grow, and this will make you more tired as well.

Headache

During the first trimester of your pregnancy, you may experience headache due to any of the following:

- Increased level of *estrogen* in the body
- Increased volume of circulating blood
- Presence of *ketone* in your system as a result of not eating enough carbohydrates and your body using fat to supply you with energy
- Stress
- Dehydration
- Hypoglycemia caused by excessive vomiting

The headache that some women experience during the last trimester of pregnancy may be the result of a condition called preeclampsia. *See Complications of Pregnancy for more information on preeclampsia.*

Treatment

Some ways to treat and prevent headaches include the following:

- Drinking at least two liters of water on a daily basis but little by little
- Avoiding caffeine, alcohol, and tobacco
- Eating little by little but regularly
- Eating enough carbohydrates to supply your body with energy
- Resting and relaxing, preferably in the dark
- Breathing deeply
- Exercising
- Going for a body massage[xi]

Stretch Marks

Stretch marks are red or pink or brown streaks on the skin. In most cases they appear on the thighs, buttocks, abdomen, or breasts.

Causes

Stretch marks are the result of the stretching of the skin during pregnancy, and in most cases they disappear after delivery.

Treatment

Apply pure tissue oil or Vaseline or glycerin to the affected areas at least twice a day.

Dry, Itchy Skin

Some women complain of dry, itchy skin around their belly and breasts during pregnancy.

Prevention and Treatment

Some ways you can avoid or treat dry skin include the following:

- Avoiding hot baths
- Using normal soap and rinsing your skin thoroughly
- Massaging the affected areas with pure tissue oil or with Vaseline or with glycerin.

Please consult your doctor if your skin's dryness and itchiness is serious and accompanied by other symptoms like dark urine, fatigue, loss of appetite, nausea, vomiting, or diarrhea as it could signal a liver problem (cholestasis).[xii]

Dark Marks

Many women notice dark spots (also known as chloasma) on their forehead, nose, cheeks, nipples, breasts, and the inner part of their thighs. They also may notice a dark black or white line, depending on their skin color, that goes from the pubis to the belly.

Causes

The change in hormonal production during pregnancy increases the secretion of melamine (a pigment that determines the skin color of an individual). These marks may disappear totally or they may simply fade after delivery.[xiii]

Treatment

Apply pure tissue oil to improve the appearance of your skin.[xiv]

Backache

Backache is a common symptom among many pregnant women.

Causes

Some of the causes of backache during pregnancy include the following:

- Change of posture during pregnancy, especially during the last trimester; also responsible for numbness and any tingling sensation in the hands and arms
- Pressure of the gravid womb on the back
- Stress[xv]

Treatment

Try any of the following methods to help alleviate backache during pregnancy:

- Sit in a comfortable chair that has a straight back, arms, and firm cushions.
- Use a footrest to elevate your feet slightly.
- Avoid crossing your legs.
- Avoid sitting for more than an hour without taking a break by walking or just standing for a few minutes.
- Stretch your back regularly.
- Avoid standing for long periods of time.
- Use your knees while bending instead of your back.
- Avoid heavy lifting.
- Avoid high heels and flat shoes; a five-centimeter heel is recommended.
- Use a firm mattress and a suitable pillow.
- Use warm or cold compresses to massage your back pain.
- Take warm baths.
- Exercise.
- Massage your back and neck.

If the pain is severe, a doctor may prescribe pain relievers. Always consult your doctor first before taking any medication during your pregnancy.

Leg Cramps

Leg cramps, or involuntary muscle contractions, may be caused by any of the following:

- Increased body mass during pregnancy putting pressure on both legs
- Gravid womb placing pressure on blood vessels that return blood from your legs to your heart
- Slow blood circulation
- Gravid womb compressing nerves that go from your trunk to your legs
- Calcium deficiency

Prevention and Treatment

The following are some helpful ways you can prevent getting leg cramps:

- Avoid standing for long periods of time.
- Avoid crossing your legs while sitting.
- Stretch your calf muscles regularly during the day and several times before you go to bed.
- Take a warm bath before bed.
- Drink enough water throughout the day but little by little.
- Take walks, but avoid getting overtired.

- Lie down on your left side to allow good blood flow in your body.
- Rotate your ankles and stretch and move your toes regularly while seated.
- Warm and massage your legs.
- Elevate your legs while sitting or sleeping.
- Take a magnesium supplement.[xvi]
- When you have a leg cramp, gently flex your toes; you will feel a sort of pain at first, but after it will relieve the cramping. Then place a warm water bottle on your legs.
  Drink milk fortified with calcium and vitamin D.
- Take a supplement of calcium and vitamin D on a daily basis if recommended by your doctor.

In severe cases of leg cramps, a doctor may prescribe muscle-relaxing drugs.

Varicose Veins

Varicose simply indicates a dilatation of the veins, particularly the veins in the legs.

Causes

The later stages of pregnancy affect normal blood flow return; as a consequence, the veins in the lower limbs enlarge. The increased volume of circulating blood in your veins weakens the valves inside your veins.[xvii]

Prevention

The following methods may help you avoid getting varicose veins during your pregnancy:

- Exercise using your legs. Marching is the best exercise for varicose veins.
- Elevate legs while sitting or lying down.
- Sleep on your left side with your legs elevated on a pillow. (This position prevents your fetus from putting pressure on your leg veins.)
- Wear elastic support stockings.
- Control your weight.
- Decrease your salt intake.
- Avoid tight clothes or clothes that may compress your waist or groin.
- Avoid standing for long periods of time.
- Avoid crossing your legs while sitting.

Treatment

The following methods will help you treat varicose veins:

- Warming and massaging legs
- Elevating legs while sitting or sleeping
- Dressing affected area using an elastic support stocking

Allergies

Hormonal changes during pregnancy increase the sensitivity of the body as well as the risk of allergies. Some allergies that may be noticed during pregnancy:

- Asthma
- Rhinitis
- Pruritic urticarial papules and plaques of pregnancy (also known as PUPPP or PEP)

On the other hand, being pregnant lowers the immune reaction of your body to allow the infant to grow in your womb. This process decreases the intensity of any preexisting allergies.

Note: Consult your medical practitioner as soon as you notice the first symptoms of an allergy.

Constipation

Constipation is the inability to have regular bowel movements. This condition is frequent during pregnancy.

Causes

During pregnancy your body produces an increased amount of *progesterone,* a hormone that relaxes muscles with a purpose to prevent uterine contractions. This hormone also affects the digestive tract and decreases bowel movements. Compression of the rectum by the growing womb also causes constipation as well as taking iron in high doses.

Consequences of constipation include hemorrhoids and a bleeding rectum.

Symptoms

The following symptoms indicate constipation:

- Lack of defecation for more than twenty-four hours
- Smaller, harder feces than usual that are difficult to release
- The feeling of having feces in the bowel when it is empty
- Bleeding rectum during defecation

- Abdominal pain and discomfort

Treatment

The following methods will help you treat constipation:

- Eating food rich in fiber
- Drinking enough water (at least two liters per day)
- Exercising

Consult your doctor if these methods do not help.

Note: Not all laxatives may be taken during pregnancy. Always consult a medical practitioner to find out which one is suitable for you.[xviii]

Heartburn

Heartburn is a burning sensation from the chest to the throat noticed after eating a meal. Many women experience heartburn during their pregnancies, and it usually starts during the second trimester of pregnancy and continues into the third trimester.

Causes

During pregnancy, the *placenta* produces *progesterone,* which relaxes the valve between the stomach and the esophagus. This situation allows acid from the stomach to go up the esophagus and give you that terrible sensation.

Progesterone also slows the wave-like contractions in the esophagus and intestines. The growing baby also places pressure on your abdominal cavity and compresses your stomach, allowing acid to go toward the *esophagus.*[xix]

Treatment

- Avoid alcohol; tobacco, caffeine; carbonated drinks; chocolates; acidic foods like citrus fruits and juices, tomatoes, mustards, and vinegar; processed foods, mint products; spicy foods; fatty foods; seasoned foods; and fried foods.
- Avoid eating big meals at once and instead eat little by little and regularly.
- Take your time to eat and chew your food properly.
- Avoid drinking a big quantity of fluid at once and instead drink little by little until you reach two liters at the end of the day.
- Do not eat close to bedtime; go to bed at least two hours after your meal.
- Do not sleep flat but instead in a half-sitting position using several pillows.
- Wear loose-fitting clothing.

- Bend at your knees and not at your waist.
- Stop smoking because it increases stomach acidity.

Avoid auto medicating, and consult your doctor for management of your heartburn.

Note: Pregnant women must not take antacids that contain aluminum.

Complications of Pregnancy

Gestational Diabetes

Gestational diabetes is glucose intolerance, which usually occurs only from the twenty-fourth week of pregnancy.

Hormones produced by the placenta may cause the insulin resistance that leads to gestational diabetes.[xx]

Symptoms

Symptoms of gestational diabetes are the same as those of diabetes mellitus for nonpregnant women:

- Thirst
- Passing urine regularly
- Feeling hungry all the time

- Tiredness
- Blurred vision

If you are diagnosed with gestational diabetes, you will be placed on a special diet. However, if diet alone does not solve the problem, your doctor may put you on insulin, as oral antidiabetic drugs are forbidden during pregnancy.

Gestational diabetes increases your risk for hypertension, heart disease, kidney disease, nerve damage, blindness, and coma.

Dangers

Having gestational diabetes can lead to your having a large baby, which can trigger some danger during the later stages of pregnancy, including miscarriage, having a stillborn child, and shoulder damage to the infant because he or she is bigger in size than the birth canal.

Many larger babies must be taken by C-section as they are too big to be delivered naturally.

Prevention and Treatment

Women who have had gestational diabetes during pregnancy have a higher risk of developing type 2 diabetes mellitus later on. To avoid developing type 2 diabetes, remember to control your weight through diet and regular exercise.

Note: Consult your doctor at the first sign of symptoms of gestational diabetes.[xxi]

Hypertension

Tension is the power or pressure that blood puts on the walls of the arteries. Hypertension occurs when that pressure is above normal, meaning the first reading or first number is higher than 140 mm of mercury, and the second reading or lower number is higher than 90 mm of mercury.

Hypertension may affect coronary arteries and cause heart disease. It may also lead to heart and kidney failure, stroke, and even death. Hypertension is also known to affect eyesight and cause poor vision.

Effects

To the pregnant woman hypertension may cause any of the following:

- Heart or kidney failure
- Preeclampsia, eclampsia, and finally death
- Damage to the liver

To the embryo or fetus hypertension may cause any of the following:

- Miscarriage

- Premature birth
- Low birth weight
- Stillborn

Prevention

To prevent hypertension during pregnancy, be sure to exercise and eat a diet low in salt and low in fat but rich in fiber.[xxii]

Preeclampsia

Preeclampsia is a condition that starts around twenty weeks of pregnancy and is characterized by hypertension and kidney failure, a condition characterized by hypertension, the presence of proteins in the urine and by swollen legs.

Preeclampsia affects the placenta as well as the mother's kidneys, brain, and liver. When preeclampsia causes seizures, the condition is then called eclampsia. If this condition is not well managed, it may kill both mother and child.

Symptoms

The following are common symptoms of preeclampsia:

- Hypertension
- Presence of proteins in the urine
- Swollen legs
- Headache
- Blurred vision
- Sensitivity to light
- Abdominal pain

Treatment

To save the life of both you and your unborn child, your doctor will plan a C-section before your due date.

Risk Factors for Developing Eclampsia

The following are risk factors for developing eclampsia:

- Women who developed preeclampsia
- Obese women
- Pregnant women under age twenty and over age forty.
- Women pregnant with twins
- Women with diabetes mellitus
- Women with kidney disease, rheumatoid arthritis, or scleroderma
- Women with chronic hypertension[xxiii]

Packing Your Maternity Bag for the Hospital

Once you reach thirty-six weeks of pregnancy, be sure to have your maternity bag packed and ready to go to the hospital. Before this time, pack little by little as you can so that hopefully you won't forget anything.

The list below can help you as you pack.

Maternity Bag Contents

For You:

- Two nightgowns
- One bathrobe
- Towel and facecloth
- Three bras
- Underwear
- Slippers and socks
- Comb and brush
- Toothbrush and toothpaste
- Soap and shampoo
- Lotion and hair products
- Deodorant and makeup
- A book or magazine
- Cell phone and air time
- Phone book and diary
- Camera

- Earphones for music
- Nail clippers

For Baby:

- T-shirts
- Caps and socks
- Baby sheets
- Baby blankets
- Diapers
- Towel and facecloth
- Baby soap and lotion
- Baby powder and Vaseline
- Baby's comb and shampoo
- Clothes to wear when discharged
- Earbuds

Part 2: Labor and Childbirth

In the following sections, we will discuss each stage of labor and how to handle delivering a child at home if necessary.

Stages of Labor and Childbirth

Labor is the process by which a pregnant woman who has reached nine months of pregnancy delivers her mature baby. It is divided into three stages:

Stage 1

During Stage 1 you will experience uterine contractions characterized by a painful sensation in your lower abdomen and lower back. These contractions, which help the cervix to thin (efface) and open (dilate) to release the child, will be regular and progressive, and they will increase in intensity. At first they will be present every thirty minutes, but with time they will become more frequent and more painful.

A creamy-white heavy vaginal discharge will come out of your vagina, and you may experience bleeding or have a watery fluid running from your vagina as well.

When you notice any of these signs, consult your nearest clinic or call your doctor or midwife for help.

Stage 1 may last over fourteen hours, particularly for a first pregnancy.

Because labor requires great energy, be sure to drink milk or juice between contractions. Do not be surprised if you vomit due to the intensity of the uterine contractions.

If at any point you are no longer able to move your legs, please call an ambulance for assistance immediately.

Remember to breathe deeply while in pain, but do not push. Do your best to relax; it is not easy, but you will manage.

When Your Water Breaks

Do not panic when your water breaks, even if it happens in a public place. Everybody can see that you are pregnant, and they will not be surprised when it happens.

Call your doctor or midwife or ask to speak to someone on the staff of the hospital where you will deliver, and tell them that your water has broken. At this point, they will most likely ask you to come to the hospital.

Place a sanitary pad in your underwear as fluid will continue flowing.

Stage 2

Stage 2 lasts anywhere from fifteen to sixty minutes. It is the stage in which the baby is born.

Contractions become stronger during this period.

If the ambulance delays in getting you to the hospital, please hold your thighs behind your knees or hold your legs against your thighs.

Stage 3

Stage 3 begins just after the baby is born and ends with the delivery of the placenta. It is a vital stage for your survival. You may feel more contractions as the placenta separates from the uterine wall.

Note: If you experience a trembling or tingling sensation during labor, it means you are breathing in too much oxygen. To stop this sensation, put your loose hand on your mouth and nose to allow you to breathe back your own air.

What to Do If the Baby Arrives Before the Ambulance

It is very dangerous to deliver alone at home, but if it happens please act as follows:

- Do not cut the umbilical cord. Instead, tie it using a clean baby sock, lace, cotton, or a peg.
- Suck gently your baby's nose and mouth using your mouth.
- Hold your baby by his or her feet with his or her head facing downward.
- Massage the baby's chest to release all secretions, if any.
- Suck again your baby's nose and mouth.
- Wipe your baby properly using a clean facecloth, baby nappy, or clean towel.
- Properly cover your baby and breast-feed him or her.
- Remain lying down on your back or on your side until the ambulance arrives.

Note: Do not try to push and expel the placenta from your womb unless it comes out by itself.

What to Do If the Baby Is Not Crying at the Time You Deliver and the Ambulance Is Delayed

- Make sure that all the fluid from the baby's lungs is drained out.
- Hold your baby by his or her legs with his or her head facing down, and blow forcefully on his or her chest.
- Remove the secretion from his or her mouth and nose.

- Put the baby on his or her side in a position where the head is lower than the body to drain out all remaining fluid from his or her lungs if there is any.
- Flick the bottom of the baby's feet strongly using your index finger to stimulate his or her respiration.
- Blow gently into your baby's nose, and massage his or her heart using your fingers.
- Repeat this process until the baby cries.

Part 3: Your Newborn

The following sections discuss your newborn's appearance at birth and how to handle certain newborn issues like jaundice, rash, allergies, fever, abdominal colic, constipation, and circumcision.

What to Expect: Your Newborn's Appearance at Birth

At birth the baby's head is larger than the rest of his or her body. On the upper front and at the back of the newborn's head are *fontanels*, or soft spots where the bones of your baby's skull have not yet grown together. This allows your child's skull to compress during labor and to grow during his or her early life.

The *frontal fontanel* closes by eighteen months but may also close earlier.

The *posterior fontanel* closes up by the second month of life.

After birth you may notice that the baby's head is swollen under the scalp; this condition is called *caput succedaneum* and will disappear after one or two days.

You may also notice an effusion of blood around the cranial bones; this condition is called *cephalhematoma* and will disappear within few weeks.

Your baby's genitals may seem to be large because of edema, but after a week they will become normal.

Your baby's eyes react to light, but they are still unable to focus on one thing.

Babies will react to noise by shaking their arms and legs (this is proof that they hear), but this is an involuntary reaction.

The newborn's stomach protrudes.

Newborn skin is wrinkled and scaly and is covered with a cheesy-like substance called *vernix caseosa*. After two weeks your baby's skin will become very dry. A white baby's skin is red, and in some cases may turn yellow. A black baby's skin is yellow at birth, but it is a bit difficult to observe the change to a darker pigment.

Newborn babies cry, suck, and sneeze.

Note: A cry at birth is a sign that the baby is alive; when a baby does not cry, it is considered a bad sign.

Newborn weight varies between 2,700 kg and 3,600 kg. Newborns from diabetic mothers may weigh up to 5,450 kg at birth.[xxiv]

Newborn Jaundice

Newborn jaundice is a yellow color of the baby's skin and other tissues of the baby's body. It is very common during the first week or two of your baby's life.

There are two kinds of jaundice: physiological and pathological.

Physiological jaundice affects 50 to 60 percent of newborns. This type of jaundice usually appears by the third day of life and may last for two weeks. In premature babies it may last up to two months of life. Physiological jaundice starts in the face then moves to the trunk and later to the limbs and extremities.

Physiological jaundice is diagnosed by sight, by blanching the skin with digital pressure, and by performing a blood test.

The causes of physiological jaundice are as follows:

- Destruction of fetal hemoglobin as it is replaced by normal hemoglobin
- Immaturity of the baby's liver so that it isn't successfully removing bilirubin from the blood
- Accidental passage of the mother's blood to the child during birth

While physiological jaundice begins seventy-two hours after birth, *pathological jaundice* begins twenty-four hours after birth and signals an extreme medical emergency.

What to Do When You Notice Your Baby Is Jaundiced

Consult a pediatrician for assessment and to find out if the jaundice is physiological or pathological.
If it is physiological, your child's pediatrician will request that you expose your baby to the sun's rays. Exposure to these rays will convert unconjugated bilirubin into conjugated bilirubin and release it through the baby's stool.

Note: For the sun's rays to penetrate your baby's skin properly, he or she must be naked, but do not forget to protect his or her eyes from sun's rays and from the wind.

Do not delay seeking medical attention for jaundice. If your baby is not helped in a timely manner, seriously complications, such as damage to the brain, can develop.

Newborn Rashes

Rashes are common in newborns. Most of the time rashes are not pathological, but some of them are.
Uncommon rashes may be symptoms of fungal, bacterial, or viral infections.

If your baby has a rash, consult his or her pediatrician for assessment and to find out if the rash is pathological or not.[xxv]

Newborn Allergies

An allergy is an immune response to an allergen.
Anything may be an allergen to anybody, but most allergies are caused by flower pollen and mold. An allergen is anything that makes your body produce *histamine* (a hormone produced by the body to protect you from anything that it considers dangerous for you).

Some babies are very sensitive to some substances. When a sensitive baby comes into contact with an allergen by inhaling, touching, or swallowing or by receiving an injection of something that his or her body considers dangerous, the baby's system will produce histamine to protect him or her from that substance.

Histamine will make your baby's body react to an allergen in ways such as having a runny nose, sneezing, coughing, experiencing shortness of breath, or experiencing itching or swelling.

For a baby, an allergic reaction may be serious and can cause death.

A baby may have an allergic reaction to certain foods, lotions, soaps, flower pollens, gases, chemicals, dust, animal fur, or mold.

Signs and Symptoms of Allergies in Nnewborns

Newborns may experience a stuffy nose, irritation of the eyes and throat, cough, or diarrhea when allergic to something in their environment.

Note: Children with nasal allergies may easily develop sinusitis, otitis (inflammation of the ear), and asthma. Consult a pediatrician for assessment once you notice the first signs of an allergy in your baby.

Prevention

To prevent your baby from developing allergies, keep him or her away from tobacco and other kinds of smoke, odor, dust, airborne pollutants, mold (avoid darkness and humidity as well as they can generate mold), animal dander, and mites.

Foods like dairy products, eggs, and nuts must be delayed until the baby is at least one year old due to high risk of allergies.[xxvi]

Fever in Newborns

Fever is an elevation of body temperature above normal. A normal anal temperature must be between 36 and 37.9°C. A temperature 38°C and above is considered fever.

Fever is a natural response of the body to infection and is often the first sign of infection, indicating that there is something abnormal in the body and that the body needs to fight against it by producing more antibodies.

Germs are comfortable with a body temperature of 37°C but uncomfortable once this temperature is above 37.5°C.

Fever is dangerous in newborns as their immune systems are still immature and unable to efficiently fight infection; also, fever may be the symptom of a life-threatening disease. **Do not forget that fever is an alarm and must be followed up to find out the cause.**

If fever does not affect your baby's behavior and your baby is still drinking, eating, and playing despite the fever, a doctor may choose not to lower the fever with medication so that the child's body may fight the infection naturally. In such a case, a doctor will request that you to give enough fluids to prevent dehydration.

Note: Do not decide on your own to let the fever clear up the infection, but always consult your medical practitioner and follow his or her instructions.

If you do not have a thermometer, you may evaluate your baby's body temperature by kissing his or her forehead or by touching the forehead using your cheek or the back side of your hand. However, using a thermometer is better as it will give you an accurate reading.

Fever is serious when your baby is less than three months old. If the baby is older than three months, fever is considered serious when it affects his or her behavior.

Note: If your baby is three months old and older and the fever does not affect his or her behavior, a doctor may request that you wait for at least twenty-four hours before consultation to allow the other signs of infection to be present and noticed, as it can be difficult to give a diagnosis with fever as the only symptom.[xxvii]

Natural Treatment Methods

The following are some natural treatment methods you can try in helping reduce your baby's fever:

- Remove clothing if the baby is overdressed.
- Give your baby a lukewarm bath.
- Put a cool wet cloth on your baby's forehead, neck, or bottom.

- Open windows, but protect the baby from wind.
- Increase baby's fluid intake by nursing more often or by giving more frequent feedings.
- If the fever is still above 38.5 °C late in the night, give a half dose of analgesic just to decrease it a bit as fever fights infection naturally.

Newborn Abdominal Colic

Twenty percent of newborns suffer from colic.

Causes

The following are a list of common causes of newborn colic:

- Immaturity of the digestive system
- Sensitivity of the digestive system
- Less gastric juice and enzymes in the baby's digestive system to break down milk
- Painful gases produced during digestion of all the nutrients he or she receives from breast milk or from formula
- Lack of bacterial flora that help in the digestion process
- Crying and screaming that makes him or her swallow air
- What you eat that gets to him or her through your breast milk

Signs of Colic

The following are common signs of colic in an infant:

- Crying anytime but especially right after a feeding
- Baby starts crying and stops immediately after passing gas or after defecation
- Frequent   spit-up
- Distended stomach
- Enlarged belly
- Pulling his or her knees to the abdomen while crying

Colic begins three weeks after birth and lasts up to three or four months later.

Babies with abdominal colic eat well and gain weight normally.[xxviii]

Protecting Baby from Colic

Identify triggers of colic and protect your baby from them.

Common triggers include the following:

- *Hunger.* Recognize all the signs of hunger and give the breast/bottle before your baby may cry.

- *Swallowing a bubble of air while crying or while sucking.* If feeding formula, check to make sure there aren't any air bubbles in the bottle before feeding. Also make sure that the hole in the bottle nipple is not too small or too large as this may make your baby swallow air. While feeding burp regularly as it will help him or her to release air bubbles. If breast-feeding, burp between switching breasts.
- *Wet diaper/nappy.* Check your baby's diaper/nappy regularly.
- *Overfeeding.* Avoid overfeeding your baby by taking notice of when he or she is full, i.e. pushing the bottle away or refusing the breast.
- *Foods or medications you are taking.* If breast-feeding, be aware that any foods you eat or medications you take are passed through your breast milk and may affect your baby's stomach.
- *Kind of formula.* Change the formula that he or she is taking as it may be the cause.

Note: If after trying to prevent colic there is no change, consult your child's pediatrician.[xxix]

Newborn Constipation

Neonatal constipation is a condition in which a child releases fewer and harder stools. Literally we may say constipation is an expulsion of small and hard stools after more than twenty-four hours. This condition makes your baby cry while defecating.

Causes

The following are the most common causes of constipation in an infant:

- Formula
  Infant formula can be difficult to digest and does not have all the ingredients found in breast milk that help to maintain baby's digestive tract. Breast-fed babies are less likely to develop constipation as breast milk contains bacteria that breaks down proteins and makes bowel movments easier.
- Dehydration
- Psychological causes
  When a child does not like to defecate, he or she contracts his or her muscles, which contracts the rectum and pulls up stools. The more stools delay in the bowel, the more they become dry and difficult to release.
- New milk or new food
- Stress
- Insufficient intake of fiber and water
- Intoxication in a case of metal poisoning
- Neurological causes
- Hormonal causes
- Malformation

Signs

The following are common signs of constipation:

- Fewer and firmer stools less than once daily
- Pain upon defecating
- Hard stools surrounded by blood
- Newborn pulling his or her legs toward his or her tummy while defecating

Treatment

We will describe two methods here to help relieve constipation in your baby.

First method

The approach described here includes natural methods you can try to help your baby with constipation:

- Give your baby a warm bath.
- Massage your baby's tummy but not his belly.
- Massage your baby's lower back and thighs.
- Pull up your baby's legs and perform a bicycle movement.
- Apply petroleum jelly on your baby's anus and gently stimulate it with a thermometer by

pushing it in and out. (Please do not go far, but just introduce less than half the size of the thermometer and do not leave it inside the anus.)[xxx]

Second method

The following approach describes other methods you can try in alleviating constipation:

- For a formula-fed baby, add an extra bottle of water when preparing a bottle.
- Change the formula only if it has been requested by a pediatrician.
- Introduce fiber into baby's diet by adding apple juice or diluted prune juice, apricot juice, peach juice, or plum juice.
- Add some drops of olive oil in baby's bottle three times a day.
- Use a glycerin suppository only if all other natural methods do not help.

If none of these help, consult your child's pediatrician.[xxxi]

Note: Breast-fed babies have many soft stools that look like seedy mustard. Formula-fed babies have fewer, firmer, and darker stools.

Later when solids are introduced, the number of stools decreases; they will become firmer, and bowel movements will become easier.

Circumcision

Circumcision is the removal of the skin (foreskin) that covers the head of a male's penis (glan).

Reasons

There are different reasons why males undergo circumcision, some of them religious, cultural, social, and hygienic/medical:

Religious: The Bible recommends all males be circumcised from the eighth day of birth.[xxxii]

Cultural: In some cultures per example In the Democratic Republic of Congo circumcision is a must. All males have to be circumcised before at least one year in age.

Social: To conform yourself to the society in which you are living.

Hygienic/Medical: Circumcision prevents phymosis. It decreases the risk of penis cancer.

Circumcision decreases the risk of STDs and HIV, but even when a male is circumcised he has to protect himself from STDs and HIV.

At What Age Should a Male Be Circumcised?

The right time for circumcision is from birth until one month; after one month circumcision becomes a more delicate procedure.

Circumcision heals more quickly in children; it does not need to be stitched, and there are fewer complications. However, a male may still undergo circumcision beyond childhood.

In some cases a doctor may delay circumcision for medical reasons:

- Prematurity of the child
- Abnormality of the penis, as the foreskin may be needed for a correctional process
- Child is sick[xxxiii]

Circumcision Complications

In some rare cases, an individual may present some complications from circumcision, including hemorrhage or local infection.
In general the circumcision wound normally heals between seven and ten days.

If there is persistent bleeding, fever, swollen penis, presence of pus or blisters on the penis, or absence of urine for twelve hours, consult a medical practitioner immediately.

Caring for the Circumcision Wound

Very carefully clean the wound using any diluted skin antiseptic liquid like Betadine (iodine) or apply Savlon antiseptic cream. You can also apply Mercurochrome or petroleum jelly.

Part 4: Caring for Your Baby

In Part 4, we will discuss how to care for your baby during the first year, including understanding your baby's cries, breast-feeding, immunizations, and how to handle issues like lactose intolerance or febrile seizure.

Lactose Intolerance or Milk Allergy

Lactose intolerance or milk allergy usually appears within a few weeks but not exactly after birth.

Symptoms

Symptoms of a milk allergy in your baby include any of the following:

- Skin rashes, such as eczema
- Vomiting
- Swelling of mouth, lips, and tongue
- Difficulty breathing, wheezing, and persistent cough
- Sneezing and runny nose
- Sinus congestion/snoring
- Watery and reddish eyes
- Frequent ear infections
- Foul-smelling stool

- Baby rejects the bottle
- Baby becomes unsettled after feeding
- Abdominal colic and watery diarrhea [xxxiv]

Treatment

Consult your pediatrician if you suspect your baby may have a milk allergy. He or she may ask you to change the type of formula you are using, or if you are breast-feeding, you may be asked to eliminate dairy products from your diet.

Understanding Your Baby's Cries

Your baby may cry due to any of the following:

- Anger
- Hunger
- Wet diaper/nappy
- Tiredness
- A need for affection/being held or carried
- A need to burp
- Abdominal colic
- Constipation
- Cold or heat
- Fear
- Distress
- A need to play

- To express that he or she is not feeling well

Crying is the only way your baby has to express himself and communicate.[xxxv]

If you feel your baby's crying is excessive and you are struggling to console him or her, consult your pediatrician.

Congenital Syphilis

Syphilis is a sexually transmitted disease caused by a germ called *Treponema pallidum*.

Congenital syphilis occurs when an infected mother transmits the disease to her unborn child. Syphilis may also be transmitted via blood transfusion or when you cut yourself with an infected sharp item like a razor blade or needle.

Symptoms

The following are symptoms of congenital syphilis in an infant:

- Inability to gain weight
- Fever
- Irritability
- Absence of nose bridge

- Blisters on palms of hands and on soles of feet
- Copper-colored flat rashes on face, palms of hands, and soles of feet
- Rashes on mouth, genitals, and anus
- Watery discharge from the nose

Children affected by congenital syphilis usually die before or just after birth.

In an older child, symptoms of congenital syphilis include the following:

- Deformity of the face
- Gray mucus from the mouth, vagina, and the nose
- Scarring skin around the mouth, vagina, and anus
- Neurological problems
- Peg-shaped teeth
- Bone pain
- Swollen joints
- Bone deformity in lower legs
- Refusal to move arms and legs because of pain
- Cloudy corneas
- Blindness
- Decreased hearing or deafness[xxxvi]

Treatment

Consult a pediatrician once you notice any of the signs of congenital syphilis.

Prevention

To prevent syphilis from spreading, consider the following:

Abstinence
Single, faithful relationship
Use of condoms
Proper antenatal care in order to diagnose and treat the disease

Febrile Seizure

A febrile seizure is a convulsion trigged by a fever. These types of seizures can happen between the ages of six months and five years.

When a baby experiences a febrile seizure, he or she may turn over his or her eyes or vomit, and his or her skin will look a bit darker than usual. Also your child's limbs may become stiff, and he or she will experience a loss of consciousness.

A seizure usually lasts a few seconds, but it may last up to fifteen minutes.

Call an emergency team once a seizure lasts for more than three minutes.

After a seizure a baby will be weak and sleepy, but in some rare cases he or she may be completely normal.

Febrile seizures do not harm children and end without treatment, but children should still be treated following the seizure as their body temperature will still be high.

In most cases seizures happen when the temperature is above 38°C, but it may also happen with a temperature less than this.

Febrile seizures can happen within the first twenty-four hours of fever.

What To Do in a Case of Febrile Seizure

- Put a child on his or her side.
- Turn the child's head to the side to prevent suffocation if he or she vomits.
- Loosen his or her clothes.
- Make sure that the child's mouth is empty, and do not put anything in the mouth during the seizure.
- Do not try to lower the fever during the seizure, but record how long the seizure lasted.
- Rush the child to the nearest hospital if he or she turns blue or if a seizure lasts for more than three minutes.

Note: Consult and report to a medical practitioner all abnormalities noticed even if the seizure lasted less than three minutes.[xxxvii]

Breast-feeding

Breast milk provides the best nutrition for your baby. It contains all the nutrients that your baby needs as well as antibodies to protect him or her from stomach viruses, lower respiratory diseases, meningitis, ear infections, some cancers, diabetes mellitus types 1 and 2, and hypercholesterolemia, among others. Even if a breast-fed baby suffers from any of these illnesses, their severity is greatly reduced.

Breast milk is inexpensive and ready at any time, and the temperature is always suitable for baby.

Breast-feeding also helps establish a connection and affection between you and your baby.

The first breast milk that your baby receives right after delivery is called colostrum, and it is rich in proteins and contains less fat than normal breast milk that your body will produce later on. It is some of the most important breast milk your baby will receive as it is full of antibodies that will help protect your baby from many diseases. Colostrum also helps your baby to release meconium, or his or her first feces.

Start breast-feeding within an hour after you deliver your baby.

The quantity of milk your body will produce is proportional to the needs of your baby. Therefore, at the beginning you will produce only a small amount of milk because your baby's stomach is still small, but you will feed your baby more frequently. As your baby grows and his or her stomach becomes bigger, your body will produce more milk to respond to his or her needs, and your baby will be able to take in more milk at one feeding and nursing sessions won't be as frequent.

Note: The more you breast-feed your baby the more milk your body produces.

Immune protection induced by breast milk lasts beyond the breast-feeding period.[xxxviii]

The following is a list of other benefits of breast-feeding and breast milk for you and your baby:

Benefits for Mom

- Breast-feeding has contraceptive effects.
- It helps to decrease stress and your risk of developing postpartum depression.
- Breast-feeding helps to stimulate uterine contractions to shrink your uterus back to its normal size more quickly after giving birth. It also helps prevent extra bleeding problems.
- Breast-feeding decreases your risk of developing breast and ovarian cancer.
- It also helps decrease your risk of developing osteoporosis later.
- Breast-feeding helps you lose extra kilograms gained during pregnancy more quickly.

Benefits for Baby

- Breast-feeding prevents allergies and obesity.
- Breast-feeding prevents constipation as breast milk contains bacteria that breaks down proteins and makes bowel movements easier.
- Breast milk has a hormone called Motilin that helps the bowels to move properly in order to release stools.
- Breast milk does not give diarrhea like other milks.
- Breast milk boosts baby's brain development.
- Breast milk boosts baby's immune system.
- Breast milk protects baby from diabetes mellitus and from lymphoma.

How to Breast-feed Your Baby

For you to breast-feed your baby properly, you need to do the following:

- Be seated comfortably.
- Put your baby on your legs.
- Put your baby's tummy against yours, his or her head facing your breast.
- Hold your baby's head with one arm.
- With the other hand, hold your areola (the colored ring around the nipple) between your

index finger and your thumb, and place the other three fingers and the rest of your hand under your breast.

- Stroke your baby's upper lip with your nipple.
- He or she will open his or her small mouth widely and grasp it.
- When your baby latches on to your breast, make sure that he or she grasps not only your nipple but a large part of your areola in his or her mouth as well; a good latch helps you to avoid nipple pain.

Do not wait for your baby to cry before you offer your breast, but give it as soon as you notice the first sign of hunger. Common signs of hunger include the following:

- Mouthing
- Increased activity
- Opening mouth and looking for your nipple
- Alertness
- Crying (which is actually the last sign of hunger)

Note: Wake your baby if he or she has slept for more than four hours and breast-feed him.[xxxix]

Diet for a Breast-feeding Mother

Eat small, regular, balanced meals, but increase your intake of carbohydrates. As a breast-feeding mother, you need four hundred to five hundred calories more than a non-breast-feeding mother.

Drink plenty of fluids, but avoid caffeine and alcohol as both pass into the milk. One cup of coffee is enough for a day.

Note: If you baby seems to be irritated, develops a rash, or has an upset stomach every time you eat a particular food, do not hesitate to remove it from your diet.[xl]

Breast-feeding Issues

While breast-feeding has many benefits, some mothers encounter problems while nursing.

Psychological problems

A breast-feeding mother may face some psychological problems, such as feeling overwhelmed by your baby and the demands of nursing in the first couple of months and feeling exhausted due to the inability to sleep properly.

Physical problems

A breast-feeding mother may experience nipple pain, engorgement, or mastitis.

In which circumstances is breast-feeding forbidden?

Breast-feeding is forbidden only in the case of some kinds of diseases like HIV; active, untreated tuberculosis; malnutrition; and breast cancer.

Complementary Foods for Baby

Complementary foods may be given to your baby beginning at the age of four months, although the World Health Organization suggests to breast-feed exclusively until the baby is six months old before introducing solids.

Baby's Diet According to Age

From six to eight months: When introducing solids to your baby (between six to eight months of age), you can begin by giving him or her soft porridge made with fortified cereals and mixed with milk two to three times per day. Choose cereals rich in iron as its level decreases from breast milk from at the age of six months.

At the beginning cereals must be watery, but with time you may make them thicker as your baby gets used to solid meals.

From nine to twelve months: From nine months give soft porridge three to four times per day. Also give your baby fruits and vegetables in the form of purées. You may use bananas, pears, apples, apricots, prunes, avocados, potatoes, and carrots.

Give some proteins, but mash them properly before giving them to your baby. You may give meat, fish, or beans. This helps prepare your baby for adult food.[xli]

How do you make purées?

Take the following steps to make your own purées:

1. Clean fruits and vegetables properly.
2. Boil them until they become soft.
3. Mash them using a blender.
4. Add milk to get the right consistency.

Immunizations

Immunizations protect your baby from specific diseases.

What Are Immunizations?

Immunizations give attenuated germs to an individual with a purpose of stimulating his or her immune system to produce specific antibodies against that specific germ.

Childhood Immunization Calendar

Birth	BCG Poliomielite Engerix-B
Six weeks	First dose of DPT + Poliomielite Engerix-B Haemophilus influenzae Type B
Eight weeks	Rotatrix PCV
Ten weeks	Second dose of DPT + Poliomielite Engerix-B Haemophilus influenzae Type B

Fourteen weeks	Third dose of DPT + Poliomielite Engerix-B Haemophilus influenzae Type B
Sixteen weeks	Second dose of Rotatrix PCV
Six months	Third dose of Rotarix PCV
Nine months	Varilrix PCV Priorix
Twelve months	Havrix Junior
Fifteen months	Prlorlx PCV
Eighteen months	Repeat of DPT + Poliomielite Energix-B Haemophilus influenzae PCV
Four to six years	Repeat of DPT + Poliomielite Prlorlx
Ten years	Cervarix (for females only)
Twelve years	TD

BCG: Vaccine against tuberculosis
Engerix-B: Vaccine against hepatitis B
DPT: Vaccine against diphtheria, acellular pertussis, and tetanus.
Rotarix: Vaccine against rotavirus
Varilrix: Vaccine against chickenpox
Havrix: Vaccine against hepatitis A

Priorix: Vaccine against measles, mumps, and rubella (MMR)
Cervarix: Vaccine against cervical cancer
TD: Vaccine against tetanus and diphtheria
PCV: Pneumococcal vaccine

Pneumococcal (PCV) is only recommended for high-risk groups ages two to six.[xlii]

Signs to Call Your Child's Doctor

The following signs should alert you to contact your child's doctor as soon as possible:

- Unconsciousness
- Stiffness of the neck
- Headache associated with limb pains
- Eye pains
- Pale skin
- Upset stomach and releasing black stools
- Upset stomach and releasing bloody stools
- Upset stomach associated with fever
- Upset stomach associated with dehydration
- Vomiting associated with fever
- Ear pain
- Fever affecting your child's behavior
- Sore throat
- Cough associated with fever
- Cough associated with vomiting

- Cough associated with bluish color on lips and fingernails
- Fever and vomiting (could signal ear infection)
- Runny nose associated with fever
- Pain when passing urine
- Generalized rash associated with fever
- Abdominal pain

First-Aid Kit

A first-aid kit is a bag containing medicines and materials necessary for rapid intervention before a patient may reach a medical practice.

It's a good idea to prepare a first-aid kit to keep in your home for emergencies you and your family may encounter.

This bag usually contains the following items:

- Spirits and other disinfectants like Savlon, Dettol, or Betadine
- Cotton wool
- Gauze
- Eye pads
- Bandages
- Elastoplasts (surgical adhesive tape)
- Scissors
- Thermometer
- Small torch

- Blood pressure machine
- Paracetamol (mild analgesic)
- Antihistamine cream

Note: This bag must be locked and kept on top of a cupboard where children may not reach it, and it must be taken wherever you are going for holiday.

Part 5: Postnatal Care

The final portion of this book details postnatal care, particularly in dealing with postpartum depression.

Postnatal Care

Six weeks after delivering and every month thereafter, you must bring your child to postnatal services for follow-up.

Nurses will check the baby's weight and evaluate if he or she is growing well or not.

They will also provide immunizations and give advice concerning your baby's growth and care.

During these visits you are encouraged to ask questions about how to take care of your baby or how to deal with specific problems related to your baby's growth.

Note: During the first visit, both you and your child will be checked.

Postpartum or Postnatal Depression

Postpartum depression is a kind of depression that 5 to 25 percent of women experience anywhere from two to four weeks after they deliver a child. Some women may experience it a few days after delivering their baby, and a third of women present symptoms from the time they are still pregnant.

Symptoms

Postpartum depression is characterized by the following kinds of feelings:

- Sadness
- Hopelessness
- Low self-esteem
- Exhaustion
- Tearfulness
- Loss of interest in things you once used to enjoy
- Anxiety
- Guilty thoughts
- Feelings of being overwhelmed
- Inability to be comforted
- Impaired speech
- Panic attacks
- Emptiness
- Suicidal thoughts
- Low mood
- Irritability

- Appetite changes
- Sleeplessness
- Tiredness
- Inability to enjoy anything
- Avoidance of people

Symptoms may disappear after several months, but in some cases symptoms may last for a year.
A woman affected by postnatal depression may struggle to look after herself, her baby, and her family.

Causes

There is no apparent cause of postpartum depression, but there are some factors that increase your risk for getting it:

- Psychological or physiological trauma related to childbirth
- During pregnancy you have a higher level of hormones, especially progesterone. After giving birth there is a sudden and sensitive decline of progesterone secretion, which, in association with some psychiatric conditions like preexisting depression; hard childhood; marital, social, or financial problems; and increased demand and responsibility, especially from the baby, places you in a position to face postpartum depression.
- Lack of breast-feeding
- Lack of social support

- Unplanned child
- The fact of having less time for yourself
- Worries about the ability to be a good mother[xliii]

Treatment: It's All about Attitude

Take the following approach to deal with and overcome this condition:

- Admit that you are undergoing postpartum depression before it becomes worse.
- Recognize that postnatal depression is a medical condition among others and that there is nothing to be ashamed of.
- Recognize that it is not your fault that you are sick because you did not choose to be this way.
- Talk to your doctor or a sister from the nearest clinic for orientation and help.
- Eat a healthy diet (a lot of vegetables and fruits).
- Drink enough fluids (at least two liters per day.
- Go for a body massage.
- Exercise.
- Get plenty of rest.
- Listen to gospel music.
- Go and consult your counselor or psychiatrist with your partner or your best friend.
- Respect the appointment with a counselor or psychologist or psychiatrist because they will help you to discover the main cause of your condition and treat it.

- Take your medications as prescribed if you are prescribed any.
- Join a support group for others experiencing postpartum depression.

Note: Alcohol worsens postnatal depression.

Conclusion

Remember that it's important for you and your partner/spouse to consult a clinic from the time you decide to conceive rather than waiting until you are already pregnant. Early planning can help identify and eliminate any diseases that could delay conception or affect the baby's growth.

Once you are pregnant, know that you are not only responsible for your life but for your baby's life as well.

Continue consulting health professionals during pregnancy until you deliver and also after for postnatal care.

---

[i] WebMD, "Is It Safe to Get Vaccinations During Pregnancy?" WebMD, June 17, 2012, http://www.webmd.com/baby/

pregnancy-is-it-safe-to-get-vaccinations.

ii BabyCentre Medical Advisory Board, "What is my rhesus status, and how will it affect my pregnancy?" BabyCentre, September 2012, http://www.babycentre.co.uk/a568837/what-is-my-rhesus-status-and-how-will-it-affect-my-pregnancy.

iii NHS Choices, "Rhesus disease," NHS Choices, November 10, 2011, http://www.nhs.uk/conditions/rhesus-disease/pages/introduction.aspx.

iv WebMD. "Folic Acid and Pregnancy," WebMD, July 29, 2012, http://www.webmd.com/baby/folic-acid-and-pregnancy.

v NetDoctor, "Ferrograd folic (ferrous sulphate, folic acid)," NetDoctor, November 22, 2011, http://www.netdoctor.co.uk/diet-and-nutrition/medicines/ferrograd-folic.html .

vi "BabyCentre Medical Advisory Board, "Vitamin D in pregnancy," BabyCentre, June 2013, http://www.babycentre.co.uk/a1023146/vitamin-d-in-pregnancy.

vii NHS Choices, "Have a healthy diet in pregnancy: Eating well when you are pregnant," NHS Choices, [date published], [website].

viii WebMD, "Foods to Avoid in Pregnancy," WebMD, May 30, 2012, http://www.webmd.com/baby/foods-avoid-pregnancy.

ix Saurace, Paul, MS, "Guidelines for Exercise: Training during Pregnancy," APA Fitness, [date published], [website].

xiii KidsHealth, "Exercising During Pregnancy," KidsHealth, November 2011, http://kidshealth.org/parent/nutrition_center/ staying_fit/exercising_pregnancy.html#.

x Wikipedia, "Morning sickness," Wikipedia, June 27, 2013, http://en.wikipedia.org/wiki/Morning_sickness.

[xi] American Pregnancy Association, "Pregnancy and headaches," American Pregnancy Association, March 2013, http://americanpregnancy.org/pregnancyhealth/headaches.html.

[xii] The Bump, "Itchy Skin During Pregnancy," The Bump, http://pregnant.thebump.com/pregnancy/pregnancy-symptoms/articles/itchy-skin-during-pregnancy.aspx.

[xiii] Academy Women's Healthcare Associates, "Skin Conditions During Pregnancy,"Academy Women's Healthcare Associates, http://www.awha.com/skin-conditions-during-pregnancy.html.

[xiv] BabyCentre Editorial Team, "Why is my skin turning darker?" BabyCentre, July 2013, http://www.babycentre.co.uk/x25007115/why-is-my-skin-turning-darker.

[xv] WebMD. "Back Pain in Pregnancy," WebMD, July 7, 2012, http://www.webmd.com/baby/guide/back-pain-in-pregnancy.

[xvi] Harms, Roger W., MD, "What causes legs cramp during pregnancy, and can they be prevented?" MayoClinic, http://www.mayoclinic.com/health/leg-cramps-during-pregnancy/AN02132.

[xvii] NHS Choices, "Varicose veins," NHS Choices, August 20, 2012, http://www.nhs.uk/conditions/varicose-veins/pages/whatarevaricoseveins.aspx.

[xviii] What To Expect, "Constipation During Pregnancy," What To Expect, http://www.whattoexpect.com/pregnancy/symptoms-and-solutions/constipation.aspx.

[xix] BabyCentre, "Heartburn in pregnancy," BabyCentre, July 2011, http://www.babycentre.co.uk/a242/heartburn-in-pregnancy.

[xx] Wikipedia, "Gestational diabetes," Wikipedia, August 2, 2013, http://en.wikipedia.org/wiki/Gestational_diabetes.

American Diabetes Association, "Gestational Diabetes," American Diabetes Association, http://en.wikipedia.org/wiki/Gestational_diabetes.

NHS Choices, "Diabetes and pregnancy: Gestational diabetes," NHS Choices, March 22, 2013, http://www.nhs.uk/conditions/pregnancy-and-baby/pages/diabetes-pregnant.aspx#close.

xxi WebMD, "Pregnancy and Gestational Diabetes," WebMD, http://diabetes.webmd.com/guide/gestational_diabetes.

xxii WebMD, "Preeclampsia and High Blood Pressure During Pregnancy," WebMD, November 3, 2010, http://www.webmd.com/baby/tc/preeclampsia-and-high-blood-pressure-during-pregnancy-topic-overview.

xxiii Wikipedia, "Preeclampsia," Wikipedia, July 30, 2013, http://en.wikipedia.org/wiki/Preeclampsia.

xxiv Discovery Fit and Health. "Appearance of a Newborn," Discovery Fit and Health, [date of publication], http://www.health.howstuffworks.com/guide/pregnancy and parenting/baby health/newborn development.

xxv NHS Choices, "Skin rashes in babies," NHS Choices, December 12, 2011, http://www.nhs.uk/conditions/skin-rash-babies/Pages/Introduction.aspx#close.

xxvi [Organization name/Author name], "Understanding your child's allergies," [Website name], [Date of publication], www.bon.airefilters.com/../child.html.

Fink, Jennifer L.W., "Allergies in Babies," The Bump, http://pregnant.thebump.com/new-mom-new-dad/baby-symptoms-conditions/articles/allergy-baby.aspx.

xxvii WebMD, "Parents' Guide to Soothing Your Crying Baby: Your Baby's Temperature and Fever," WebMD, March 3, 2012, http://www.webmd.com/parenting/baby/crying-colic-9/temperature-fever.

Miller, Ayala, MD, "Top 10 things pediatricians want you to know about your newborn: Newborn fever," FoxNews.com, www.foxnews.com/Health/2012/03/26/t.

BabyCentre Medical Advisory Board, "Fever," BabyCentre, February 2011, http://www.babycentre.co.uk/a84/fever.

[xxviii] Lawrence, T.A., "The cause and treatment of newborn, infant, and baby colic,"Colic Calm.com, www.coliccalm.com/ baby_infant_newborn.

[xxix] MedlinePlus, "Colic and crying," MedlinePlus, August 8, 2011, http://www.nlm.nih.gov/medlineplus/ency/ article/000978.htm.

[xxx] NetDoctor, "Baby constipation (Reviewed by Dr. Patricia Macnair)," NetDoctor, November 21, 2011, http://www.netdoctor.co.uk/health_advice/facts/babyconstipation.ht m.

[xxxi]Hoecker, Jay L, MD, "What are the signs of infant constipation? And what's the best way to treat it?" Mayo Clinic, http://www.mayoclinic.com/health/infant-constipation/AN01089.

[xxxii] Holy Bible, *Genesis* 17:10-14.

[xxxiii] Ripton, Nancy, "When's the best time to circumcise?" Just the Facts Baby, www.justthefactsbaby.com/Pregnancy/.

The Circumcision Decision, www.thecircumcisiondecision.com/.

[xxxiv] Himamshu, "Signs of formula allergy in your newborn baby," Unicef, January 22, 2013, www.babycare.onlymyhealth.com/ signs.for.

xxxv Dubinsky, Dana, "Twelve reasons for baby's cry and how to soothe them," BabyCentre, www.babycenter.com/home/baby /carringand colic/why babies cry.

xxxvi MedlinePlus, "Congenital syphilis," MedlinePlus, December 1, 2011, http://www.nlm.nih.gov/medlineplus/ency/ article/001344.htm.

xxxvii NHS Choices, "Febrile seizures," NHS Choices, [date of publication/review], [website].

KidsHealth, "Febrile seizures (reviewed by Yamini Durani, MD)," KidsHealth, July 2012, http://kidshealth.org/parent/ general/sick/febrile.html.

xxxviii BabyCenter Medical Advisory Board, "Breastfeeding: Getting Started," BabyCenter, http://www.babycenter.com/ 0_breastfeeding-getting-started_465.bc.

Wikipedia, "Breastfeeding," Wikipedia, August 6, 2013, http://en.wikipedia.org/wiki/Breastfeeding.
xxxix Wikipedia, "Breast milk," Wikipedia, July 18, 2013, http://en.wikipedia.org/wiki/Human_breast_milk.

Breastmilk.com, http://www.breastmilk.com/.

American Pregnancy Association, "What's in Breast Milk?" American Pregnancy Association, January 2013, http://americanpregnancy.org/firstyearoflife/ whatsinbreastmilk.html.

xl Mayo Clinic Staff, "Infant and toddler health: Breast-feeding nutrition: Tips for moms," Mayo Clinic, http://www.mayoclinic.com/health/breastfeeding-nutrition/MY02015.

BabyCenter Medical Advisory Board, "Diet for a healthy breastfeeding mom," BabyCenter, http://www.babycenter.com/

0_diet-for-a-healthy-breastfeeding-mom_3565.bc?page=1.

[xli] World Health Organization, "Complementary feeding," World Health Organization, http://www.who.int/nutrition/topics /complementary_feeding/en/.

[xlii] Just Mommies, "Children's immunization schedule," Just Mommies, http://www.justmommies.com/Justmommies/Health.

[xliii] Wikipedia, "Postpartum depression," Wikipedia, July 27, 2013, http://en.wikipedia.org/wiki/Postpartum_depression.

Mayo Clinic Staff, "Postpartum depression," Mayo Clinic, http://www.mayoclinic.com/health/postpartum-depression/DS00546/TAB=indepth.

PubMed Health, "Postpartum depression," US National Library of Medicine, September 19, 2012, http://www.ncbi.nlm.nih.gov/ pubmedhealth/PMH0004481/.

www.ingramcontent.com/pod-product-compliance
Lightning Source LLC
Chambersburg PA
CBHW070750290526
45795CB00002B/551